thought HAS NO CALORIES

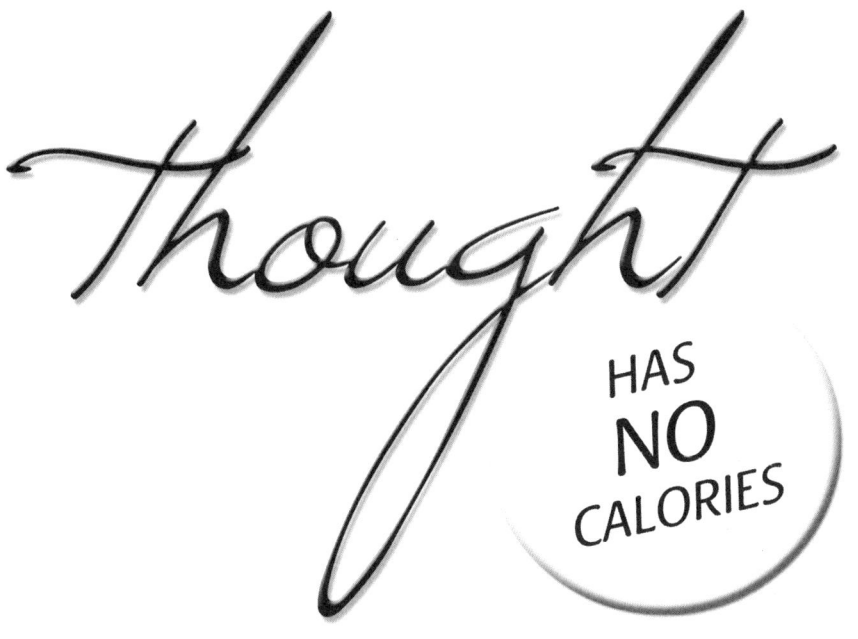

Mind Nourishment:
The ONE MINUTE Diet Remedy

Lynne Lambert

Advantage

Copyright © 2008 by Lynne Lambert

All rights reserved. No part of this book may be used or reproduced in any manner whatsoever without prior written consent of the author, except as provided by the United States of America copyright law.

Published by Advantage, Charleston, South Carolina.
Member of Advantage Media Group.

ADVANTAGE is a registered trademark and the
Advantage colophon is a trademark of Advantage Media Group, Inc.

ISBN: 978-1-59932-070-0
LCCN: 2008926314

Most Advantage Media Group titles are available at special quantity discounts for bulk purchases for sales promotions, premiums, fundraising, and educational use. Special versions or book excerpts can also be created to fit specific needs.

For more information, please write: Special Markets, Advantage Media Group, P.O. Box 272, Charleston, SC 29402 or call 1.866.775.1696.

Table of Contents

Section One – Why I Wrote — 7

YOUR INVITATION TO CHOOSE	11
YOU ARE A CREATOR	12
SOURCE OF STRENGTH	18
CREATING YOUR NEW TRUTH	21
TEN NEW OPTIONS FOR THOUGHT	25
THE SACRED ACT OF DIETING	41
THE ONE MINUTE DIET REMEDY	45
THE MIND NOURISHMENT RECIPE	50

Section Two – Daily Reflection — 55

MY WORDS OF PROMISE AND COMMITMENT	55
DAILY REFLECTIONS	58-176
Thirty Mind Nourishment Statements	
Thirty Today's Body Miracles	
Thirty New Motives	
Thirty Active Choices Charts	
Thirty Personal Perspectives	

Section Three – Nutrition Reference — 179

REFERENCES	218
MIND NOURISHMENT CARDS	219

Section One
Why I Wrote

Sometimes, our most astounding gifts in life are unveiled, only if intentionally sought.

This truth came to light for me after many years of soul searching and self-reflection. The painful consequences of the naive choices I made in my youth led me to a life altering realization – in spite of my resistance to its truth:

I AM THE CREATOR OF MY LIFE RESULTS.

That's it. In the end, I am responsible for the good, the bad, the joy and the ugly in my life today. Yes, its true that situations sometimes present themselves in a manner I would not consciously choose. Still, my life's results develop from how I respond, how I cope and how I live. Choosing to shed my excuses, blame and resentments from the past opened a world of possibilities and joy in the NOW.

The biggest shock in my journey toward this enlightenment was to admit that the greatest teachers in my life were my mother and father. My perception of their impact on my life shifted from the reason for my despair to the reason I am accountable and open to all the joy in life. Contrary to how I felt as a young adult, I now see their influence as one of my greatest blessings.

Dad was a man who lived for beer, cigarettes and golf. In that order! His distorted priorities in life were the catalyst for abandoning his wife and four little girls. Intoxicated on his ego and alcoholic beverages, he had no comprehension of the devastation he left behind or the joy he missed out of, with a family he never knew.

I spent most of my childhood yearning for a relationship with this man, but as an adult I realized I barely knew him and I wanted an adult perspective. After twenty years of no contact with him, I arrived at his doorstep only to find a weak, elderly stranger with a sour disposition. At that moment, the hope that he would fill the vacant spot I felt since childhood, dissolved. Unlike the image of the savior I had in my mind, he seemed… oh so human. This was the man I had craved all these years? All of a sudden, my yearning for his love and approval ceased. I no longer felt like a victim of abandonment. In that moment, I had clarity about personal accountability and I knew I had no control of, or blame for the absence of a father. Two months after our visit, he died of cancer, still never knowing his children. My father's priorities never made sense to me, but the day I faced him, I realized they didn't make sense to him either.

SECTION ONE - WHY I WROTE

He helped me realize that the choices others make in life are part of their unique path. His choices were personal and had nothing to do with my being lovable or worthy. With an adult perspective, I understand this man was immature, disconnected from his heart, and incapable of accepting responsibility. Whatever his issues were, I am certain they had nothing to do with me. However, the pain and confusion his choices inflicted on me as a child, drove me to find my own path and inner strength. His absence and neglect for his family helped me to develop accountability for my choices, actions and life results. The only thing I can change about the past is my perception of it. Today, it's my choice to perceive this experience as a purposeful gift.

Mom perceived the experience quite differently. After her husband left, she struggled to feed, clothe and shelter her children while dealing with a heart so heavy she could barely function. Her upbringing and religion taught her to stay in a marriage regardless of the situation. Alone, heartbroken and overwhelmed with responsibility, she looked for comfort and escape from her unbearable reality. Alcohol and drugs were not an option for her, nor would she ever leave her children at home alone to go out and find adult companionship. She felt like an abandoned prisoner in her own home. She was craving her husband, yearning to be loved, and starving for relief from a relentless pain in her gut.

Late night TV offered some distraction for her mental grief, but the pain in her gut continued. In her nightly search for comfort, she found a friend in rocky road ice cream. It was always there. It soothed her pain. It filled the void in her gut. It offered temporary distraction and relief from her agony. It anesthetized her.

Each night she sat in front of the TV watching Johnny Carson while eating her ice cream. She found this method of consoling herself so effective that it became her habit during the day as well. Not only did it numb her emotional pain, but the padding she created around her body served as a shield against anyone else who might cause her more pain. Food became her escape, her protection, her reward, her drug, her life. She didn't have to contend with the emptiness in her heart as long as she kept her gut filled.

Unfortunately, this method of comfort had severe consequences. At 5'3" and nearly 400 pounds, her body became a prison instead of the temple it was meant to be. She suffered the effects of high blood pressure, high cholesterol and diabetes. Obesity, disease and the amputation of a leg confined her and profoundly limited her ability to enjoy life.

I spent a lifetime watching my mother destroy her beautiful body with food, in an attempt to avoid her emotions. Although I am genetically prone to develop diabetes and the other physical problems she endured, my observation of her physical creation became my motivation to look deep within myself for a solution. I realized I could easily follow in her footsteps if I didn't learn how to create a different outcome for my life.

Both my parents, though unknowingly, taught me well. Their actions were gifts that positioned me to open my mind to intentional methods of creating my life. I resolve to: Find it, feel it, forgive it and move on. That is how I grow. That is how I heal – and healing is an inside job

I wrote this book for all who seek to nurture their body, expand their mind and align with their internal Spirit.

YOUR INVITATION TO CHOOSE

This book will guide you to focus on a whole-being approach to healthy living and healthy eating. Perceptions, thoughts, words and state of mind become an intentional creation, resulting in new life patterns. Here you will find guidance to create an elevated state of mind where your dieting struggles inevitably dissolve.

At the back of this book you will find 30 Mind Nourishment Cards. Cut these cards out along the perforated lines. Starting with Day One, keep one card with you each day for thirty consecutive days. Before each meal, snack or beverage, simply read a Mind Nourishment Card. At the end of each day, turn to the page in "Daily Reflections" that coincides with that card. Your unique insights and motives at mealtime are revealed as you consider these questions and research the information requested. Your creative power will be apparent to you as you become enlightened and conscious of your thoughts, words and actions.

Calculate your daily needs with the formulas provided in "Nutrition References" in Section Three. Fill in the goal boxes on each day's Active Choices Chart prior to beginning this program. Take the time to record your exercise, water and energy intake each day on the Active Choices Chart intending to match your pre-established goals.

Now, you have an educated, attainable daily goal, a motivated mindset and all the information required to make wise choices. You have it all!

YOU ARE A CREATOR

Your perfect body weight is your conscious creation every day. With the tools in this book, there are no more excuses, depression or frustration about losing or gaining weight. Now, you have the missing piece in the puzzle of dieting and you know the truth about your role in creating your life results. It's no longer a secret!

Shift your thoughts

That's it. That's the secret to creating the body weight you desire. It sounds easy, right? Well, it will be with the guidance you'll find here. YOU have the final word in creating your perfect body weight.

You are much more than flesh, bones, organs and cells. You are the miracle of Life Energy, occupying a magnificent mass of physical matter. You have the power to recreate your life with a shift of thought. This power will emerge when you accept your authority and acknowledge your creative ability. Your body responds to your mind because the intelligence of life energy extends into every inch of it. Mind and body are united as one creative expression of life, making you a creator! You are a miracle of life energy in action! Imagine your potential in life as you learn to purposely direct this powerful force.

There is no diet or therapy that can give you a consciousness of accountability and contentment regarding your body, without your willingness to shift your thought process. The incentive and formula needed to achieve your best physical and mental state is initiated with your awareness and gratitude. When you nurture and nourish your body from this state of mind you are using your creative, powerful mind deliberately. Your personal best will soon become so natural and effortless you will be better positioned to attend to the joy of living, instead of stressing about your weight. Your body is intended to be an asset in your life journey, not a deterrent. Its purpose is to provide an environment for you to live your life in service to your spirit and in harmony with your soul's purpose.

Your journey in life is unique and cannot be compared to others. Your goals will be specific to your individual needs. If you are currently dealing with a physical challenge, its origin or reason may be a mystery to you. We are all human and subject to human conditions. We all seek answers and healing for our physical challenges and the feeling of being powerless that accompany these unwanted conditions. Often, it is our feeling of being powerless that prompts us to turn to a higher source of power for solace. Whatever your situation, your creative word, your attitude and how you choose to focus your attention always has an impact in your life. Regardless of your past, today you have the power to choose perspectives that will initiate improvements in your experience of life.

The health industry has provided ample information about the quantity of healthy food to choose for dieting success. Body weight problems aren't due to lack of available support and guidance. Anyone who has failed at achieving and maintaining their desired body weight knows there is more to dieting success than just having information about quantities and choices of food. With so much knowledge available why is such a large portion of the population dissatisfied with body size, shape and weight? How do you initiate and sustain the drive to take advantage of effective methods of dieting? Successfully creating and maintaining a healthy body weight will evade you if you don't know how to stay conscious, accountable and knowledgeable about your body. Your mental outlook is what determines your actions and creates a physical outcome.

My client, Beverly, is an example of someone who lost her healthy perspective about food. She lives a very blessed life. The success she achieved in her job provides a constant agenda of exciting business luncheons and dinner events. Her social calendar is quite busy as well. There is not a day that passes without an invitation for dinner from one of her many girlfriends or male suitors. Opportunities to feast in the best restaurants in town consistently provide fabulous dining experiences. Beverly's popularity allows her the "good life." Whether she is conducting business or socializing with friends, her schedule always includes fine dining, exquisite wines and decedent deserts.

Her actions at mealtime were mindless as she enjoyed her abundant life. Excessive eating and drinking became an everyday occurrence as part of her social interaction and comfort. Beverly hadn't considered the devastating effect this behavior would have over a period of time. When I met Beverly she was a beautiful woman in her early forties. In spite of her infectious smile and charm, she was struggling with her bodyweight and a self-image of disgust and frustration.

Unfortunately, over time, her extravagant life style resulted in an extra seventy pounds on her beautiful body. Those extra pounds were the catalyst for her grief and low self-esteem. Depression set in every morning when she tried to get dressed and none of her clothing fit properly.

Beverly loved her life, her job and the social events available to her. She didn't want to give up her lifestyle but she knew something had to change. Her eating habits, the action that's purpose is to support life, was destroying her body and her happiness.

Her awareness and deliberate thought process at mealtime was the first thing she needed to develop. With the use of Mind Nourishment Cards she learned to take a moment before putting food or drink into her body to create a mindset of accountability and gratitude. She also took the time to chart her goals at the beginning of each day on the Active Choices pages found in this book. This provided a premeditated plan for how she intended to nourish her body on that day. She learned to separate the joy of *connecting with friends and social interaction from substance.* Her new mindset taught her how the two can coexist when she stays conscious of her actions, obtains knowledge about balanced nutrition and demonstrates respect for the abundance in her life. She had a mental and physical plan each day, each meal.

Beverly quickly regained her confidence and authentic sense of self. She still enjoys her abundant lifestyle, but her choices about food begin with a moment for reflection and an expression of gratitude regardless of where she is or whom she is with. This is now her way of life…her new habit.

Once she adapted a mindset of accountability and gratitude at mealtime, the extra pounds on her body began to disappear. Beverly now dresses in the morning with ease and comfort. She feels confident and beautiful from the inside out. Her transformation was initiated with a simple shift of thought at mealtime.

Your life results begin with the mindset you choose. Yes, you can choose! Learning to deliberately shift your thinking one day at a time, one meal at a time, will help you create a permanent state of being that supports your dieting goals for life. The influence your thoughts have in your life become clear when you look at some of their effects. Have you ever been so angry you felt your head was going to explode? Have you ever been so deeply hurt, you were certain there was a knife in your heart? These are extreme examples of physical responses to your thoughts. These responses occur on many different levels, some quite obvious and others, subtle enough that you might not realize they are affecting your everyday choices. Your daily thoughts can become an unconscious habit with undesirable impact – preventing you from making choices that support your dieting goals. It is your mental habits that dictate your physical actions and reactions. Your mind and body work in unison.

Regardless of your current habits, you can learn to deliberately direct your intentions and thoughts, enabling you to create new habits and the body weight results you seek.

> *"Thoughts become things...*
> *choose the good ones!"*
> *– Mike Dooley*

You are the only one choosing your thoughts. Take a moment to consider how much impact your thinking has in your day. Does your choice of thought encourage your best or clutter your mind and distract you from your goals? You are initiating your actions and creating your perception of reality through your thoughts and self-talk. This is your birthright and method of creation. New life creations are initiated by choosing new, purposeful thoughts and making them habitual. Stay conscious and choose thoughts of accountability and gratitude at mealtime and create your *now experience now*!

Throughout time, we have searched for the "magic pill" that achieves our desired fitness and diet goals. The "magic" can be found by searching within yourself and shifting your thinking. Look to keep your thoughts and intentions focused on your goals, rather than on your regrets. Open yourself to new perceptions and choose thoughts and words from kindness and respect toward all life (including your own). Fearful and demeaning thoughts about yourself and others dissolve when your focus is on love, peace, empowerment and faith. Access to a higher frequency of energy in life is yours when you choose to lift yourself into it. In this elevated mindset, your personal best will emerge and become a natural way of life. Now, you will know your body as a precious temple for life and you will recognize the power of your creative contributions.

> *"The significant problems we face cannot be solved at the same level of thinking we were at when we created them."*
> *– Albert Einstein*

SOURCE OF STRENGTH

There is a divine Source supplying every cell in your body with LIFE. This Source is the presence of pure light and love. Each of us experiences a unique perception and relationship with this presence and the variety of titles attached to it will depend on religion, heritage, or belief systems. The title you choose to name this Source is part of your individual path in life. The true value is not realized by the title you choose, but in the acknowledgement of your connection to an omnipresent creative Life Force. Its magnificence is illuminated by your growing knowledge and acceptance of it as the source and essence of all life. It is constant, unchangeable, limitless and ever-present. As you expand the knowledge and awareness of your connection to this Infinite Power, the inherent divine qualities within you will become apparent. Creativity, love, beauty, peace, compassion, gratitude, intelligence and intuition are natural characteristics of your being, and when expressed, they are a gift to everyone. In fact, the world relies upon your individual capacity to develop these traits in your unique way, apply them in your own life, and share them with humanity. By doing so, you raise your consciousness in to alignment with this Source and contribute to raising the collective consciousness of the world. You have been given the freedom and power to be a consciously creative human being!

You are a magnificent creation, a unique expression of life energy. Your essence cannot be duplicated. As life energy permeates every cell of your body, it causes your heart to beat and provides you with the capacity to think, feel and choose. It is no less than divine intelligence – God, Goddess, Universal Power, and Life Energy in action! Living with this knowledge at the forefront of your mind will enrich your experience of life and illuminate a path toward physical, mental and spiritual enlightenment.

> *"There are only two ways to live your life.*
> *One is as though nothing is a miracle.*
> *The other is as if everything is."*
> *— Albert Einstein*

You are a multi-faceted being, always growing and changing in mind and body. When both aspects, mind and body, are nurtured, you will be inspired to fully express the magnificence of your existence and contribute a higher purpose in life. You are a powerful creator and the only one in charge of your development. With the information provided here and a little effort on your part, you will launch a lifetime of automatic behavior for dieting success. Your knowledge and gratitude will become a constant foundation of cause to care about your creative actions at mealtime.

Although the essence of the Life Energy you embody is eternal and unchangeable, the physical body *is* changeable. If negative perceptions and emotions run rampant, they can wreak havoc on your health. When your perception of a situation makes you feel lethargic, stressed, over-anxious, fearful, or depressed, toxic chemical reactions and detrimental physical responses to those reactions occur. Consequently, your health, fitness and body weight can become an expression of your state of mind.

The good news is that, with a short time of concentrated effort, you can permanently shift to new perceptions that will eliminate the poisonous effects of negativity. You can choose to perceive life as an exciting learning experience that is always presenting new opportunities, instead of clinging to perceptions that cut you off from life. How are your perceptions serving you today? Is your method of thought a habit that enriches your life, or imprisons you? Your perceptions may be nothing more than a bad habit you can easily change by assuming command of them. Research suggests that new habits can be formed in as little as twenty-one days. This is a relatively short commitment for changes that will improve your life so drastically. You can apply the formula of new thought, new perceptions, new action and new results to any aspect of your life. You are the creator of your habits.

Recognizing and exploring the power you possess to create new, healthy thoughts can be fun and exciting. It will also be easy, once you embrace the techniques provided in this book. You will manifest a happier, healthier experience for yourself in mind and body when you intentionally SHIFT YOUR THINKING.

CREATING YOUR NEW TRUTH

Many of the beliefs that create your perceptions and state of mind have been adopted, unconsciously, over time. As a child, you may have accepted the ideas your parents, teachers and culture told you, without question. Social circumstances may have dictated your religion, ideas of acceptable behavior, your self-worth and even your opportunities in life. This belief system originated from outside sources and became your truth, quite possibly, without internal examination. Through repetition, you have become conditioned to accept the ideas of others as the truth of your being. If you learned from others to appreciate yourself as a magnificent creation of life, with the capacity to creatively express yourself, you have truly been blessed. However, if your current "truth" consists of anything less than joy, love and beauty, both in mind and body, perhaps it is time to discover a new truth about yourself. Your attention and focus can create a "truth" that will empower, enlighten, and celebrate the life gift within you.

Life graciously provides you with many gifts, one of the most valuable being free will. It is free will that allows you to create experiences in life through your choices and actions. Success, in all areas of your life, springs from accepting responsibility for your choices. The dietary choices you make are initiated by your perceptions, thoughts and words because they are the catalyst for your actions. By choosing to replace negative assumptions and degrading self-talk with empowering thoughts and words, you initiate a shift in consciousness. Open your views. Be receptive to new perceptions, new opportunities and new creations. Just as your current perceptions and creations were established by previous input, you can shift your focus and create peace and productivity with new input. You have the power and freedom to choose. Your conviction and positive, life-giving choices will build momentum. Now, you will create a new truth that will manifest your desired transformation.

> *"Whether you think you can,
> or you think you cannot, you are right."*
> — Henry Ford

Anita is a childhood friend of mine. I recall that, in the seventh grade, she repetitiously made degrading comments about herself. She often talked about how fat she was, how she wasn't pretty, wasn't smart... the wretched list went on and on, and at the time, none of this was true. I have observed this negative self-talk as a common method, used by teenage girls, to diffuse any petty jealousy that confronts them. Somehow, they think it makes them more approachable when they appear humble. At thirteen years old, our distinction between humble and self-sabotage can be skewed.

Unfortunately, Anita never learned to change her self-talk. Thirty years later she was still degrading herself. Over a course of three decades the repetitive, negative self-talk became her reality, and she packed on an extra sixty pounds. What she feels for herself is far from beautiful, and her believe of inferiority has limited her in every aspect of life. She convinced herself at a very young age that she was destined to fail.

I convinced Anita to use the Mind Nourishment Cards as an example of what a new language and self-image might feel like. Initially, she was quite uncomfortable with self-praise and also with taking responsibility for her creations in life. In her mind, she believed none of it applied to her! It actually made her laugh in disbelief, but fortunately she was willing to humor me and diligently use her cards at mealtime.

After seven days, Anita noticed a shift. She became conscious of her degrading self-talk, and learned to stop herself when she began to speak negatively. Her perspectives and motives were clarified in her evening guided-journaling. She was shifting to a new truth and developing a new sense of self. As she intentionally chose awareness and gratitude, she shed her false beliefs of inferiority. She began to take accountability for her life creations. With time and consistency, the extra pounds disappeared and have not returned. In fact, her purposely created mindset has improved every aspect of her life!

Your perceptions invoke thoughts. Your thoughts stimulate feelings, and it is these thoughts and feelings that determine your choices and actions. When it comes to your fitness, attempting to reshape your body, without reshaping your belief system, is like trying to change an effect without considering the cause.

You have inherited a creative capacity from your Creator. It is your choice of thoughts, words and actions that dictate your experiences, and such can be utilized as a formula for achieving your desired body weight. Assume the command to direct your creative capacity by nourishing your mind with positive, life-supporting perceptions and beliefs. Your results are yours to consciously create when you realize the magnitude of your power to think positively and act decisively.

"The definition of insanity is to repeat the same actions and expect different results."
— Albert Einstein

Your gifts in life include an unlimited array of untested ideas, actions, and results. The only requirement is that you open your mind, and then move in the direction of your desires. You are standing on the threshold of new possibilities with every new moment. If what you're thinking and doing is not producing your desired results, I invite you to nourish your mind by exploring your options. The following ten new options for thought will initiate a receptive state of mind and assist you with your desired life results.

TEN NEW OPTIONS FOR THOUGHT

1. Expand Your Awareness and Create an Empowered State of Mind

Life is constantly moving, changing, and expanding. Don't allow yourself to miss out on the joy of *now* by becoming stuck in the events of yesterday. When you decide to trust and enjoy the process of life, your decision will allow you to be comfortable, even enthusiastic about the dynamics of change. It is your nature to move, transform and expand, in the infinite possibilities of the universe. If you're not willing to realize and appreciate the joy in the moment, you could become a victim of your past experiences, and stagnate mentally and physically.

Know that you possess the power and the courage required to live in a state of awareness, open to joy and success. This empowered state of mind will direct you toward your desires. Look deep within and realize the power to create this state lies inside you! It's been there since birth. Remember your childlike wonder and fearless exploration? You are by nature, a joyous being. Call upon that joy again.

Expanding your awareness and purposely returning to your natural state of empowerment could be the missing link when seeking physical transformation. It is your choice to embrace responsibility for supporting regeneration of your body. Physical changes begin with entertaining new thoughts, choosing a new life-affirming vocabulary to describe yourself and adapting your belief system to these new ideas. As your mind changes, your body will also change. Self-motivation is a natural state when you purposely shift your thinking towards the positive action you wish to manifest.

Your life is important in the grand scheme of creation! You are a ray of light that is part of the great light of humanity. You complete the universe. Begin by knowing this truth and utilize it to motivate yourself.

> *"We ourselves feel that what we are doing is just a drop in the ocean. But the ocean would be less because of that missing drop."*
> *— Mother Teresa*

Expanding your mind becomes easier as you make room for the present by letting go of issues from the past. Choose to live in the present and allow the freedom of being in the NOW. Your mental state at this very moment determines how you view reality. Being stuck, being weighed down by old emotional wounds is cumbersome and oppressive to our minds and bodies. Choose to let it go. Travel light. Seek a gift in every situation, and a gift will reveal itself.

Conscious Creation Exercise Suggestions:

Meditate for at least fifteen minutes each day.

In your daily vocabulary, replace the phrase "I should" with "I am," or "I will."

Smile and say "Hello" to someone you've never met.

Observe life's simple miracles: Watch a sunset, stop and smell the flowers, or marvel at a child's way of life.

2. Entertain New Ideas of Self-Love

Self-love doesn't imply an inflated ego, nor does it imply that you believe you are more important in the scheme of creation than any other human being. I am suggesting that you create a state of mind, which is so peaceful and full of love, that it enables you to freely give love to others. Staying strong and balanced allows you to develop the traits required to give care to those you love. Caring for others is a gracious act, when motivated by love. However, if this care means neglecting your own body, mind, and spirit then you'll eventually deplete your energy. If you are sidelined by physical illness or mental exhaustion, you're not going to be the asset you wish to be in life. Sometimes our perception of what others need is just an unconscious avoidance of our own personal issues. You can give your joyful best to the world when you exude the love and peace achieved from nurturing yourself first.

Become open to new ideas of self-love by embracing the truth about the magnificent life force you are. Take time for yourself to meditate, exercise, and enjoy the beauty of nature. Love and demonstrate respect for your body by providing it with life-giving foods and physical activity, and most importantly, choose a peaceful state of mind.

Know that you are a unique and significant expression of life, requiring your loving attention. You are worthy of a joyful life, but embracing joy is your responsibility. Joy is an active principle, not a passive one. If you don't completely love yourself and honor your needs, you won't fully experience your capacity to truly love others. **You cannot give what you don't have.** You have an important purpose and a unique mission in this life. Loving yourself is an unselfish act that demonstrates gratitude for your precious gift of life. It will be this self-development that will expand your capacity and sensitivity to help others.

*"To love oneself is the beginning
of a lifelong romance."*
– Oscar Wilde

Conscious Creation Exercise Suggestions:

List at least ten reasons why you are worthy of self-love.

Make a list of simple acts that would demonstrate self-love and increase your capacity to give to humanity. Here are some examples: exercise, eat healthy, meditate and donate.

3. Take the Physical Action Needed for Accomplishment

Action is the key word here. Your thoughts and words cause movement in your consciousness. However, to accomplish your goals, your willingness to take physical action is required. Claim your divine authority to create your results in life by choosing motivating thoughts, speaking with words that strengthen your determination and taking constructive action. This is the complete formula for changing your life.

> *"Nothing happens until something moves."*
> *– Albert Einstein*

Without your physical action, there is no physical result. Are you waiting for someone else to act for you? Sorry, but that's not going to happen in most aspects of your life, including your health, fitness and diet. Your desired results occur only through your movement! Your thoughts and words are powerful; however, they are only the initiating point of your actions. Assess your participation and daily contributions to your goals and accept the responsibility required for accomplishment. You must take physical action to achieve physical goals.

Utilize the power of your combined thoughts, words and actions to reinvent your fitness level or any other aspect of your life right now.

Conscious Creation Exercise Suggestions:

Take some time right now to congratulate yourself for taking the action to read this book. A pat on the back each time you take constructive action will encourage you to take action again. Even baby steps in the right direction are an action toward your goal.

4. Acknowledge Your Creative Capacity and Use It Wisely

You have been crafted with the capacity to create. Wherever you are right now, look around at your creations. Have you planned a peaceful setting in which to read? Do you have a room in which you have created a comforting décor? Have you created and nurtured fulfilling relationship with others? What state of mind do you possess right now? How was it created?

Not only do you have the capacity to create in all the different aspects of your life, you are always creating! It's impossible to live your life and not create. Now, you can learn to direct your creativity intentionally. You have the authority to eliminate havoc, chaos or misery and create a bright and fulfilling way of life. Consciously or unconsciously, you continuously experience the effects of your powerful creativity. Your current scenarios are the outcome of your creations from the past.

Your future creations will reflect the action you take right now. Respecting and nurturing your creative capacity will readily produce your desired outcomes now and in the future.

If you have a garden and you want to grow tomatoes, you're not going to plant carrot seeds. You plant tomato seeds. With time and nurturing, the laws of nature will produce a ripened tomato. Thoughts are like seeds, and thus the same universal laws apply. If you want to create a healthy and beautiful body, you won't do it by planting seeds in your mind that tell you, "I'm fat and too old to change." You produce your desired results by planting thoughts that promote a body reflective of your enlightened sense of life. Think of your mind as a fertile garden waiting for your choice of seeds to be planted. Just as the soil in a garden needs to be fertile, so your mind must be receptive. Just as a garden needs sunlight and water, the garden of your mind needs conviction and faith.

"It's kind of fun to do the impossible."
– Walt Disney

Conscious Creation Exercise Suggestions:

Take some time to sit down and decide exactly what you would like to create in life. Write your desired creations on a card expressing your gratitude as if they already exist for you.

Example: "I am so grateful for my lean, fit, healthy body." Place the card where you will see it. Read your words aloud several times each day. Act as if you expect your desire to become a reality. Stay focused on what you wish to create.

5. Keep Your Words Constructive and Positive

Once you begin to understand the creative power of your words, provoked by your intentions, you will feel the value of expressing yourself from a positive and loving state. You are always contributing to a truth in your life with this creative power. If you think and speak in negatively about yourself or others, you are participating in and contributing to an undesirable creation in your life. Yes, your words are a powerful force and you bear the responsibility for their impact. The laws of cause and effect are impartial. All the energy you radiate is a creative force that attracts like energy unto itself, eventually returning to you. If you are investing your creative energy on bad seeds you don't want to harvest, stop contributing to their nourishment with your thinking, speaking, and beliefs.

> *"Better than a thousand hollow words,*
> *is one word that brings peace."*
> *– Buddha*

Remember, you are not separate from your Life Source. At the core of your being lie the inherent qualities of the image and likeness of God. Instead of degrading a life so precious, use the power of your own free will to elevate yourself in to a closer reflection of that image and likeness. Choose thoughts, words and actions that move you in the direction of your desired life creations. You have the power to do so!

Conscious Creation Exercise Suggestions:

At the top of a sheet of paper, write the words, "My New Life Creations." Carry this sheet of paper with you all day. Each time you discover yourself using a degrading comment to describe yourself or others, revise it. Write it down in a positive version to create a new language for your new way of approaching life.

Example: Degrading comment – "I'm too old and too tired to start something new now." Replace this statement with "New experiences keep me energized and youthful."

Each time you find yourself using the old comments, consciously revise it by choosing an empowering replacement.

6. *Forgive*

Walls of misery that block joy in your life, dissolve with forgiveness. Anger, resentment, guilt, and hatred create a toxic environment for your mind and body. Searching for, or holding on to blame for past events in life, depletes your energy and poisons your consciousness. As long as your outlook is poisoned, you can't see opportunity or experience joy. By forgiving and releasing the events of the past, you will begin to receive the soothing gift that only forgiveness can provide – peace. Forgiveness is the antidote for the dis-ease that anger, resentment, guilt and hatred produce. Your forgiveness initiates healing in your life.

To forgive yourself is to accept that you are on a spiritual path, learning about yourself and life through your experiences each day. Triumphs, as well as mistakes, are a natural part of being human. Perceived failures for actions you regret can provide new insights and be used as a gauge for situations you now know how to avoid. It has given you the wisdom to determine your intentional direction in life. Forgive yourself for your mistakes and move forward.

*"Anyone who has never made a mistake
has never tried anything new."
– Albert Einstein*

To forgive others does not imply you condone their actions or that you need to continue a relationship with them. However, it does illustrate your willingness to relinquish any pain you may be harboring in your mind caused by their actions. To be unforgiving punishes you more than anyone! The ill effects of any toxic emotions will dissolve with forgiveness. You are only responsible for your own actions, responses and reactions. If you seek opportunity in every situation to gain wisdom and a stronger bond with your Creator, this is exactly what will occur.

*"Learn from the mistakes of others.
You can't live long enough to
make them all yourself."
– Eleanor Roosevelt*

To forgive the past is to acknowledge the influence that events have upon your life. Find a gift or lesson in it, and then allow yourself to move into the present. There is no value in holding on to negativity from the past except to realize how much it limits you. Consider defining the word "forgive" as "for-gift to myself." The gift in it is always yours.

> *"The weak can never forgive.*
> *Forgiveness is the attribute of the strong"*
> *— Mahatma Gandhi*

Conscious Creation Exercise Suggestions:

Is there anyone in your life you are angry with or feel resentment toward? If so, take the time right now to send a prayer or a blessing to this person. Consciously relinquish any ill feelings you are harboring. Turn it over to a higher source of love.

Say this serenity prayer out loud when you complete your blessing: "God grant me the serenity to accept the things I cannot change, the courage to change the things that I can and the wisdom to know the difference."

7. Relinquish Any Attempt to Control Others

Keep your attention on your own personal growth and allow others to be responsible for theirs. Though in the end you each seek peace, happiness, and answers in life, you all have the right to choose different paths. The road you choose to reach your destination is unique. You'll find yourself with more time to honor your own path by learning to allow others their personal choices. Your help, support and counseling are of value when given with love. However, your purpose on this planet is not to control or manipulate others into a mold you design. This is a waste of your precious energy and shows a lack of respect and understanding for the unique path of others.

Trust that life has a divine plan for you. You move toward this plan at your own pace and in your own time. This is true for others as well. Give and be what you want to receive in life. If you want to be loved, love. If you want to be accepted, accept others. If you want to be forgiven, forgive. This demonstrates your active role in handling your own experience of life, for which you are responsible. Trust the process of life. You don't always see the bigger picture, especially in the lives of others. When your energy is focused on a higher purpose in your own life, you will shine as an example of purposeful living and your support and opinions will be sought and valued by those who are ready to receive them.

"Example isn't another way to teach,
it is the only way to teach."
– Albert Einstein

Conscious Creation Exercise Suggestions:

Take the time to process your reactions to those who condemn or judge you for your actions and beliefs or attempt to change your life in a way that doesn't feel right to you. Send a blessing to them and choose compassion in your communication with others. When you are given an opportunity to share your wisdom, respond from a place of love, not from ego. Accept and appreciate the diversity of mankind.

8. *Focus Your Attention on Gratitude*

The areas, to which you give attention, are the areas in which your life will flourish. Gratitude is a magnetic force attracting more of what you are grateful for. The sooner you realize the power your perceptions and attention play in your life, the sooner you'll be set free. The world around you will be revealed as one that enriches, not limits, your life experiences. Each experience then becomes an opportunity for growth and expansion. Infinite possibilities expose themselves, once you accept that your teachers and lessons in life come in many forms. Seek to discover the good in all. Trust in yourself, in humanity and in the goodness of life.

> *"Men are not disturbed by things,*
> *but the view they take of things."*
> *— Epictetus*

Even with all the difficulties and challenges life deals us, there are always so many gifts for which to be grateful. Express your gratitude to your loved ones and to your Life Source everyday. Find something to be grateful for in every situation.

Make a lighthearted game out of it, if you want. Gratitude will become a way of life that just might be your healing light.

Conscious Creation Exercise Suggestions:

Sit down with a sheet of paper, a pen and a timer. Set the timer for three minutes. During those three minutes, write down everything you have to be grateful for. Do not stop writing for the entire three minutes, even if you repeat yourself.

When you read what you've written you may discover a new-found sense of gratitude.

9. Manage Your Time Wisely

Time is one of our most valuable commodities. If you feel robbed of time for peace, joy, and self-reflection, you may need to do some soul searching to determine your true priorities in life. Consider how *you* might be the one who is robbing yourself of this time. Learning to set boundaries for your commitments and obligations is a crucial ingredient of wise time management. Overextending yourself can create feelings of resentment and chaos in your life, and you'll slowly lose sight of your true self. You can heal this self-created cycle of being pulled in too many directions, by learning to purposefully arrange your time. You are the choice-maker in your life. You govern your experiences in life when you choose to take responsibility to do so. By prioritizing and delegating your precious time, you will experience the joy of living in harmony with your soul's purpose. Telling yourself and others you do not have time to